50 NATURAL WAYS TO
DETOX

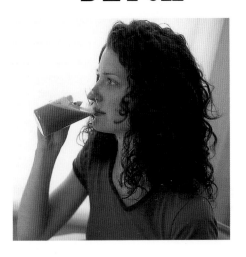

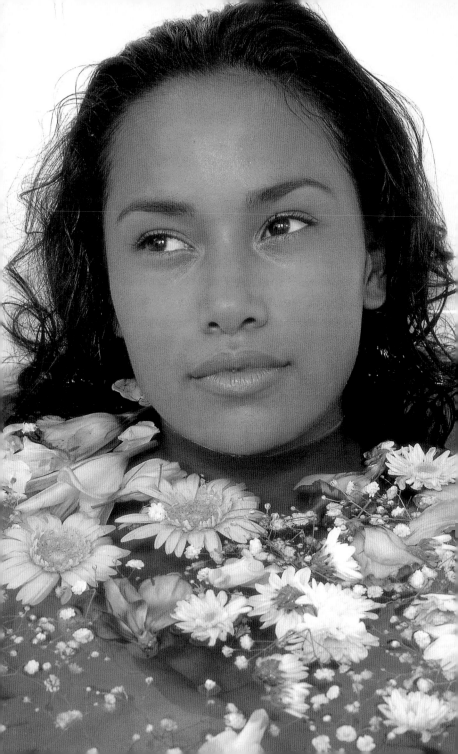

50 NATURAL WAYS TO
DETOX

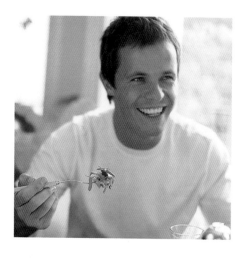

**Tried-and-tested tips shown
in over 100 photographs**

Tracey Kelly

LORENZ BOOKS

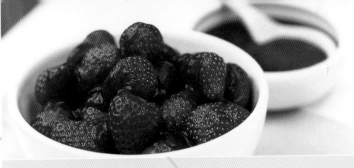

contents

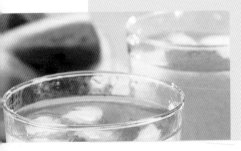

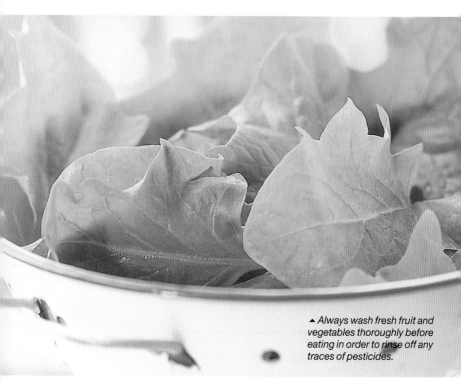

▲ Always wash fresh fruit and vegetables thoroughly before eating in order to rinse off any traces of pesticides.

introduction

In the course of our hectic lives, it is easy to overlook the longer term view of health. Under stress, we may succumb to bad habits such as smoking, drinking too much alcohol, eating too much or too poorly, and neglecting to exercise or sleep.

These factors, taken singly, may challenge the body so that its performance levels are low; two or more factors may have serious health implications over the years.

Sometimes it is a good idea to sit back and take stock of the situation. Perhaps you have had one too many colds or bouts of flu this season, or

your energy levels have fallen, so that even simple, everyday routines have become something of a struggle?

Maybe you have become all too dependent on eating junk food instead of nourishing meals, and have noticed the pounds creeping up – or just a general dullness to your skin, hair and nails? Or perhaps you've stopped exercising and your fitness levels have fallen, leaving you feeling out of shape and depressed? You know you must do something to rectify the situation, but are unsure of where to begin. This book aims to help you make a fresh start.

detox diet

By following a brief detoxification programme, you can help to eliminate harmful substances from your body, clearing the way for a healthier lifestyle and new diet and fitness goals. A detox diet, which you can plan yourself, consists of eating only a few types of unprocessed food for a short period of time, while drinking plenty of water and herbal teas. This has the effect of flushing harmful toxins out of the system, restoring your energy levels and giving you a "clean slate".

For a brief introduction to detox, try a regime that lasts only one or two days. This will ease your body gently into a cleansed state, and is ideal in that it causes few side effects. A week-long detox is more intense and should be aimed at resolving more deeply embedded problems.

If at all possible, take the week off from work and responsibilities, as the change of food, drink and routine may leave you with temporary side effects. You may experience headaches, dizziness and stomach upset as toxins are washed out of your system, but they will subside once you begin to ease back into a normal, healthy diet.

essential exercise

Also crucial to any detox regime is exercise – it stimulates the lymphatic system, gets the heart pumping and improves circulation, removing waste matter and oxygenating the cells. Not only does exercise tone the muscles, it also acts to elevate your mood by releasing chemical substances called endorphins, which will help you to cope with stress more effectively, long after you have finished exercising. Choose from a range of aerobic exercises – those that push the heart rate up, such as cycling, running and dancing – and anaerobic exercises, those that help build muscle tissue and bone density through short bursts of activity. Examples of these

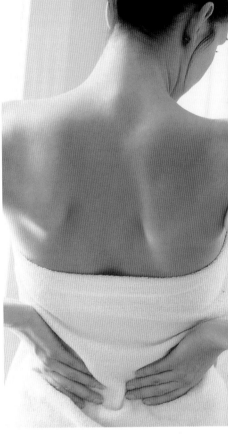

▲ Self-massage is a wonderful way to relax the body during detox, helping to ease tensions and release toxins from the cells.

are weight lifting and squash. Varying your routine will work all the muscle groups and keep you interested.

food for the soul

Relaxation and clearing the mind of negativity are just as important as physical exercise. The body and mind are fully linked – so stress, anger and negative thoughts can play havoc with your immune system, reducing its ability to eliminate toxins and making you more vulnerable to infections and disease.

By practising meditation and relaxation techniques for just 15-30 minutes a day, you will notice a marked improvement in your resilience to viruses, tension headaches and other stress-related illnesses. They will give you the ammunition to fight the daily battles that everyone is subject to – and savour life's pleasures even more.

With visualization techniques, it is possible to "rehearse" future stressful situations by imagining an important interview, for example, and then creating the conditions or solutions for a successful outcome. You can also explore what you really want from a relationship, friendships, job, home and family life.

alternative therapies

Like regular exercise, complementary therapies such as massage and aromatherapy have a beneficial effect on the lymphatic system, helping to flush out toxins. Massage has the added benefit of loosening tight muscles and helping to resolve chronic problems

▸ *Drink plenty of water throughout the day to keep you hydrated and to help your body flush out toxins.*

where tension is held in a certain area, such as the shoulders or abdomen.

Learn and practise self-massage techniques, and you will experience fewer problems with aching joints, neck tension and back pain. You can massage areas such as the face, hands and feet for an instant lift. Massaging the hands will also help you to avoid problems such as repetitive strain injury, a common hazard associated with manual and office work. Using aromatherapy oils in massage intensifies the experience.

Aim to look after your body now, and you will have less of a need to detox in the future. In addition, you will age in a more healthy way, with fewer of the complaints that beset many older people.

luxurious spa treatments

While you are following a detox regime, spa treatments such as saunas, mud wraps, body scrubs and baths will leave you feeling pampered and your skin feeling refreshed.

Saunas and wraps work by drawing impurities out of the skin, leaving the skin glowing. Other treatments such as facials, body scrubs and floral baths, are deep cleansing, mood enhancing and – best of all – enjoyable. Treat yourself by booking an appointment with a professional practitioner, or try one of the homemade treatments in this book.

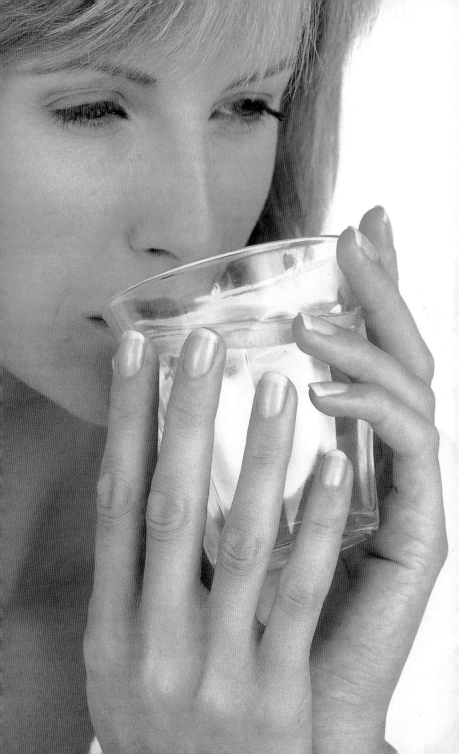

detox treatment.

This book is organized so that you can choose the foods, detox plans, massage, exercises and treatments that will assist you on the road to a healthier body and a happier mind. Create a self-tailored detox programme by eating foods that will help your body to cleanse itself: fresh fruits and vegetables; tasty nuts and grains; soothing herbal tisanes and tangy smoothies. Decide on one of four detox plans, from a revitalizing 1-day detox to a 7-day detox – a sort of "spring clean". Massage techniques will address chronic problems – for example, aching shoulders or stiff neck – and chapters on exercise and meditation describe ways to recharge the batteries, both physically and mentally. Finally, pampering spa treatments – from invigorating body scrubs to floral-scented facials – will leave you cleansed, energized and looking as fresh and beautiful as you feel.

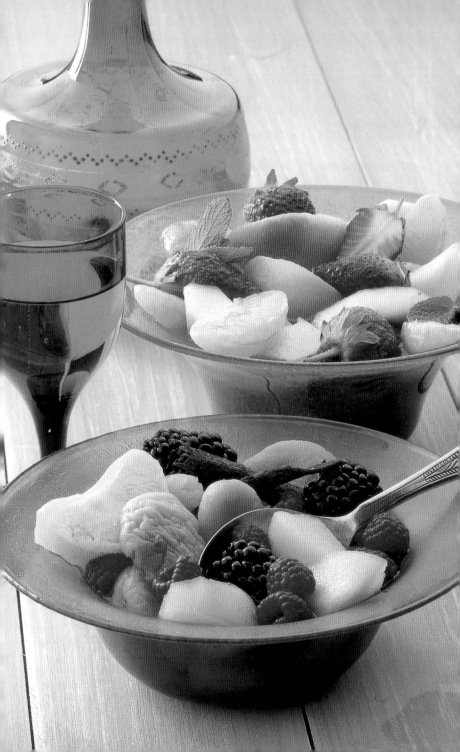

1 refreshing fruit

Fresh fruit is a storehouse of essential nutrients. Packed with vitamins, minerals, fibre, amino acids and enzymes, raw fruit should feature in any detox regime, as it helps bind and flush out toxins.

citrus fruits

These refreshing fruits are loaded with vitamin C, a powerful antioxidant that protects the body against harmful free radicals and inhibits premature aging. Antioxidants also help to reduce the risk of cancer and heart disease, and increase iron absorption.

Lemon is perhaps the best cleanser; its astringent and antiseptic properties stimulate the liver and gall bladder. A glass of hot water with freshly squeezed lemon juice is the ideal way to begin a detox day. Freshly squeezed oranges and grapefruits stimulate the digestion and tone the system. They are also an excellent source of betacarotene, calcium, phosphorus and potassium.

apples, pears and grapes

Crunchy apples contain malic and tartaric acid, which act to boost the digestive system and cleanse the liver. Their high pectin content binds heavy metals, such as lead. Apples also provide a steady stream of energy via fructose, a natural sugar.

When eaten regularly, pears help foster a good complexion and glossy

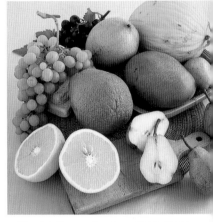

▲ The rich fibre and water content of tasty fruit make it the perfect internal cleanser.

hair. They are also an effective diuretic and laxative. Popular for one-day mono-diets, grapes are one of the most effective detoxifiers – in addition, they have been shown to relieve constipation and help kidney, liver, digestive and skin disorders. The white or red varieties are best.

mangoes

These fragrant soft fruits are reported to cleanse the blood. They also benefit the kidneys and digestive tract.

2

healthy dried fruit

Dried fruit provides plenty of sustaining energy and is invaluable in a detox regime. Although higher in calories than fresh fruit, unlike chocolate and sweets, dried fruit is a great source of nutrients.

Whenever buying dried fruit, look for unsulphured fruit, especially if you suffer from asthma. Choose from dried hunza apricots, figs, dates, raisins, apples, pears and peaches. Alternatively, you could opt for some more exotic fruits, such as pineapples, mangoes and papayas. These add tasty variety to your diet.

▾ *Perfect for snacks, dried fruit provides all the essential nutrients in a compact form.*

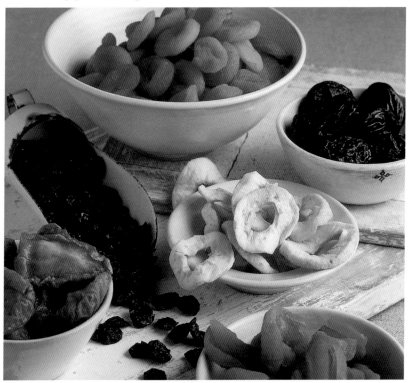

3 nutritious vegetables

The therapeutic benefits of fresh vegetables are due to an abundance of vitamins, minerals, bioflavonoids and other phytochemicals. Include plenty of different vegetables in your detox regime.

carrots

These root vegetables are highly beneficial. As well as cleansing, nourishing and stimulating the whole body, their abundant supply of betacarotene has been found to reduce the risk of cancer – eating just one medium-sized carrot per day can halve the risk of lung cancer.

garlic and onions

Containing antiviral and antibacterial nutrients, these vegetables are said to cleanse the system, fight cancer and lower blood cholesterol. Garlic boosts

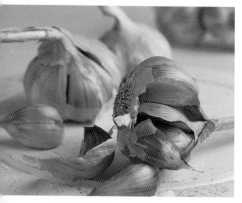

▲ *Garlic is one of the oldest-known and most potent of healers.*

the immune system and acts as an anti-inflammatory. Onions are best eaten raw, but their healing properties are not all lost through cooking.

beetroot

A powerful liver cleanser, beetroot (beet) is beneficial to the blood and a good laxative. It also has high levels of betacarotene, calcium and iron.

cruciferous family

Members of this family – including broccoli, Brussels sprouts, cauliflower, cabbage and watercress – are all among the detox superfoods. They stimulate the liver and supply a cancer-fighting cocktail of phytochemicals.

Broccoli also offers a plentiful supply of many B and C vitamins, in addition to minerals such as calcium, folic acid, iron, potassium and zinc.

spinach

A vast supply of antioxidants makes raw spinach an excellent choice for a detox diet. It contains betacarotene, vitamin C, calcium, folic acid, iron, potassium, thiamin and zinc. Young spinach makes a tasty addition to salads.

4 detox vegetable stock

Vegetable stock is used to add flavour to dishes such as soups and stews. Purchased stock is usually very high in salt, and should not be used in detox, as salt increases water retention.

veggie deluxe stock

15ml/1 tbsp sunflower oil
1 potato
1 carrot
1 celery stick
2 cloves of garlic (peeled)
1 sprig of thyme
1 bay leaf
few stalks of parsley
600ml/1 pint/2½ cups of water
freshly ground black pepper

1 Scrub, trim and chop the vegetables. Heat 15ml/1 tbsp sunflower oil in a large saucepan. Add the potato, carrot and celery, all chopped up into small pieces.

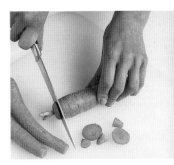

2 Cook them, covered, for 10 minutes until soft. Stir in the garlic, thyme, bay leaf and parsley. Pour the water into the pan and bring the mixture to the boil.

STOCKING UP
Larger quantities of stock can be made and stored in the freezer, or in the refrigerator to be used within 4 days.

3 Simmer the mixture, partially covered, for 40 minutes. Strain, and then season with freshly ground pepper. Use the vegetable stock as required in cooking.

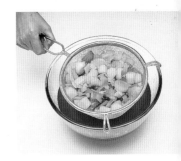

5

wholesome grains

Not only are whole grains and cereals an excellent source of low-fat protein, they contain complex carbohydrates, fibre, vitamins and minerals to keep you energized during detox.

world of grains

Grains have been a part of the human diet for thousands of years, and have been cultivated for centuries. It is good to include a selection of different grains in your detox plan, including brown rice, barley, millet, oats, couscous, buckwheat and quinoa. Brown rice is used to treat digestive disorders, calm the nervous system and reduce the risk of bowel cancer. Oats absorb impurities in the blood, leaving the complexion glowing. The South American grain, quinoa, contains more protein than any other – about 14 per cent.

essential fibre

Unprocessed whole grains contain both soluble and insoluble fibre, both of which are fundamental in the prevention of constipation, colon and rectal cancers, ulcers and heart disease. Foods rich in fibre bind with harmful cholesterol and help it to pass through the body for elimination.

wheat warning!

Although nutritionally viable in its whole form, wheat is also a common allergen – it can irritate the body's ability to absorb some nutrients, and should be avoided during detox.

◀ *The starch in grains is absorbed slowly, keeping blood sugar levels even – important when you may be eating less than usual.*

6 vital pulses

Providing low-fat protein, fibre and vitamins, beans and pulses have long been a staple of vegetarian diets. They are bursting with minerals, including folate, iron, magnesium and potassium.

bean choice

It is preferable to use dry beans in cooking, as processing adds sugar and salt. The night before beginning a detox programme, try eating a nutritious stew or thick soup made from tasty lentils, dried peas, pinto and mung beans, or chickpeas.

bean feast

Most dried beans need to be soaked for at least 8 hours prior to using them in a recipe. To prepare, leave them overnight with plenty of fresh cold water. The next morning, drain and rinse the beans before boiling hard for at least 10 minutes, then leave them to simmer until they are fully cooked. (Note: lentils do not need to be soaked, nor boiled rapidly.)

Alternatively, follow a recipe for cooking instructions. Never eat beans raw or partially cooked, as they may cause an allergic reaction. When using a new bean, taste a small amount first, in case you are sensitive to it.

▸ *Studies show that eating just half a cup of cooked beans regularly reduces cholesterol levels by 20 per cent.*

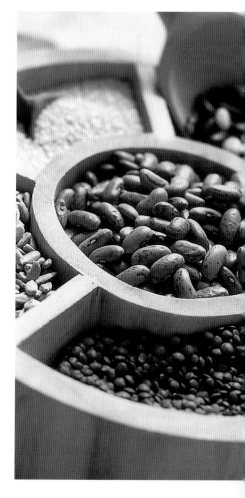

7 supersprouts

When beans, seeds and grains sprout, their nutritional value soars making them excellent detox ingredients: their vitamin C content rises by 60 per cent, and B vitamins by 30 per cent.

grow your own

It is simple to grow delicious sprouts. Commercial sprouter packs are available from health food stores, and they can be easily grown at home. Try the following:

Take a large, wide-mouthed jar and wash thoroughly. Place 15ml/1 tbsp of alfalfa seeds, soy, mung or other beans in the jar.

Cover the mouth of the jar with a clean piece of muslin (cheesecloth) or finely-woven mesh, and fasten tautly with an elastic band or a clean piece of string. Rinse the beans or seeds thoroughly in cold water, shaking off the excess. Place the jar in a darkened cupboard, and rinse the beans once or twice a day, as before.

The beans should sprout and be ready to eat in approximately 4–5 days. Once they are fully sprouted, refrigerate your supersprouts. You can keep a ready supply by beginning new jars on successive days.

▼ Sprouts supply rich amounts of protein, vitamin E, potassium and phosphorus – all packaged in an easily digestible form.

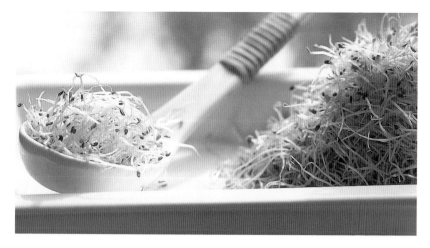

Packed with vitamins, minerals and **antioxidants,** seaweeds – such as arame, kombu, hijiki and wakame – improve the **condition** of your **skin,** hair and nails.

9

beneficial nuts & seeds

An excellent alternative to meat and cheese, protein-rich nuts and seeds are said to reduce the risk of heart disease and cancers. Their vitamin E content improves the skin, hair and nails.

nutty choice

Walnuts, almonds, cashews, hazelnuts and peanuts offer some of the best health benefits – they can be eaten on their own, or added to porridge, breads, casseroles and salads. Since they are a high-fat food, nuts should be eaten in moderation.

Seeds such as pumpkin, sunflower and sesame offer similar nutritional values with slightly fewer calories. Buy them in small quantities, seal and store in a cool place. Wholegrain toast spread with tahini (crushed sesame seed spread) makes a tasty and nutritious start to the day.

nutty oat snack

30ml/2 tbsp sunflower oil
30ml/2 tbsp honey or maple syrup
600g/21oz jumbo oats
50g/2oz sunflower seeds
50g/2oz pumpkin seeds
50g/2oz roughly chopped almonds,
    hazelnuts or unsalted peanuts
50g/2oz chopped dried apricots
    or raisins

Preheat oven to 150°C/300°F/Gas 2. In a large pan, heat the oil and honey until the mixture is thin. Stir in the remaining ingredients, except the apricots, until the dry ingredients are coated evenly. Spread the mixture on a baking sheet and toast for 30 minutes, until it turns light golden brown. Remove from the oven and stir in the apricots. Store in an airtight container.

▲ Nuts are packed with B vitamins, iron, calcium, magnesium and potassium.

10 fresh herbs

Herbs have a cleansing effect on the system, easing indigestion, nausea and constipation; they may also help to alleviate headaches and respiratory problems.

Although herbs are low in nutritional value they have a high concentration of essential oils, many of which are antioxidant, antiviral and antibacterial.

cooking herbs

Some of the most useful herbs for cooking delicious detox meals are also the most common. Look for fresh coriander (cilantro), basil, dill, mint, parsley, sage, rosemary and thyme. Many grocery stores and nurseries sell growing plants – fresh is best.

SUPER HERBS

The following cleansing herbs can complement your detox programme. Always consult a qualified naturopath before taking them for the first time.

MILK THISTLE – increases liver efficiency.
ECHINACEA – boosts the immune system.
GOTU KOLA – diminishes cellulite.
GOLDENSEAL – aids digestion and is antibacterial.
DANDELION – a gall bladder and liver tonic.

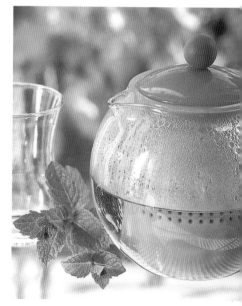

▲ Mint is a useful herb for easing nausea, indigestion and respiratory problems.

soothing mint tea

This tea is useful for your detox plan – it will settle stomach upsets and clear your sinuses. Place 10ml/2 tsp of fresh peppermint or spearmint leaves in a pot and add boiling water. Cover and leave for about 10 minutes to infuse, then strain and drink.

11 stimulating spices

Revered for their medicinal properties for thousands of years, spices are also a culinary mainstay. When added to dishes and drinks, they tend to have a stimulating and antiseptic effect on the body.

detox spice rack

Useful spices to include in your detox plan include fenugreek, nutmeg and turmeric, as they cleanse the body and help to release toxins. Cinnamon is also an effective cleanser; cardamom calms indigestion, as does coriander.

Cloves contain both antiseptic and anaesthetic qualities – clove oil has traditionally been used for toothache. Pepper is the most commonly used spice in the West. Black and white pepper aid digestion and help dispel wind, and cayenne promotes

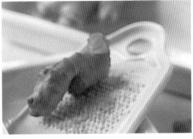

▲ Add grated ginger to salads and stir-fries.

sweating and the release of toxins through the skin (but is best used in small amounts only).

ginger

Fresh root ginger is one of the most powerful healing spices to include in a detox diet. Not only does it treat gastro-intestinal complaints and nausea, it also reduces the risk of some cancers. Add to stir-fries or grate into salads. You could also try this soothing tea: take two or three fine slices of ginger and place in a mug; add boiling water and infuse for 5-10 minutes. Add a teaspoon of honey if desired.

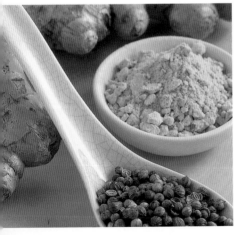

◀ Fresh root ginger, fenugreek and coriander seeds are powerful system cleansers.

12 relieving oils & vinegars

Oils provide essential fatty acids and vitamin E, both beneficial for the heart and skin. Cold-pressed oils are most nutritional. Cider vinegar is best for detoxing – it relieves headaches and aching joints.

wide choice

Organic olive, sunflower, safflower and grapeseed oils are all beneficial. Speciality oils such as walnut, sesame, almond and hazelnut are a tasty alternative. Almond oil is also good for massaging and moisturizing your body – it is easily absorbed into the skin.

Because oils are a high-calorie fat, it is important to use them in moderate amounts only during the latter days in a week-long detox diet. Wine vinegars should be avoided in detox, as they contain acetic acid, which hinders digestion.

sesame ginger dressing

120ml/4fl oz/½ cup cider vinegar
15ml/1 tbsp grated fresh root ginger
120ml/4fl oz/½ cup water
250ml/8fl oz/1 cup sunflower oil
10ml/2 tsp honey
15ml/1 tbsp sesame seeds

Place the vinegar in a bottle or jar. Add the grated ginger and allow to soak for 30 minutes. Add the water, oil, honey and sesame seeds. Shake well and add to green or fruit salad.

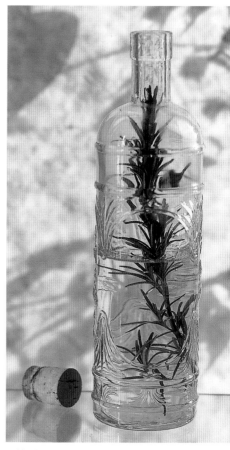

▲ Use herbs, such as rosemary, to make tasty aromatic oils for salad dressings.

13

hydrating water

Water is a vital nutrient that cannot be stored in the body. It is lost constantly through sweat, urination, defecation and exhaling vapour when you breathe. Aim to drink at least 1.5 litres/2½ pints each day.

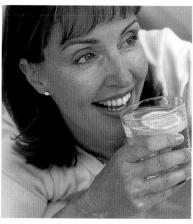

stay hydrated

Pure water – mineral or filtered tap water – will flush toxins from your organs. Diluted fruit and vegetable juices are also good choices. Avoid soft drinks containing sugar and preservatives as these place stress on your body and add sodium and empty calories. Carbonated water is acceptable, but drink it only in small amounts – dieticians believe that it raises the pH level in the stomach, making it harder for the body to digest protein.

▶ *Ice-cold water with a slice of lemon will boost your metabolism and burn calories.*

◀ *A cup of hot water with a slice of lemon is a refreshing and cleansing tonic.*

monitor your intake

It is a good idea to drink a large glass of water when you wake up in the morning, as your body dehydrates during the night, especially during warm or hot weather. It is best not to rely on your sense of thirst to tell you when to drink: keep sipping it throughout the whole day.

Most people do not drink enough fluids during the day, and this becomes noticeable when the urine turns a tell-tale dark amber colour. A pale golden colour means that you are probably taking in enough hydrating fluids.

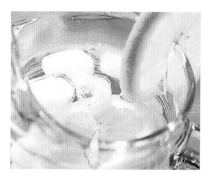

14 soothing herbal teas

Herbal teas offer medicinal benefits and, as drinks, have the advantage of hydrating the body. Unlike black teas and coffees, which contain caffeine, they do not strain the cardio-vascular system.

digestive tea

The fennel and caraway seeds in this tea aid digestion. It can be taken as a pleasant drink after a heavy meal or to soothe an upset stomach.

Put 5ml/1 tsp fennel and 2.5ml/½ tsp caraway seeds into a pot, adding 600ml/1 pint/2½ cups of boiling water. Steep for 10 minutes and serve with a dollop of honey.

bedtime tea

For a relaxing and calming tea to ease you to sleep, place 5ml/1 tsp chamomile, 2.5ml/½ tsp of valerian and 5ml/1 tsp of peppermint into a pot and infuse. Strain, add honey if desired, and drink. This is best taken 30 minutes to 1 hour before bedtime.

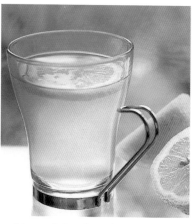

▲ A tea made from lavender and vervain helps ease the effects of overindulgence.

morning–after tea

This is a good liver reviver to take following a party or late night out. Sip it throughout the day until you feel your body and mind are refreshed. Place 5ml/1 tsp vervain and 2.5ml/½ tsp lavender flowers into a pot. Add 600ml/1 pint 2½ cups of boiling water, cover and steep for 10 minutes. Strain, add lemon and sweeten with honey.

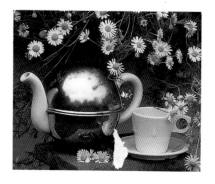

◀ Chamomile is a herb with calming, relaxing properties, perfect for bedtime.

15 flower tisanes

Teas made by steeping fresh sprigs of flowers in boiling water are called tisanes. Many blossoms can be used, such as chamomile, dandelion, lavender, rose, lime blossom, jasmine and bergamot.

lemon verbena tisane

This refreshing, lemon-flavoured tisane is delicious when enjoyed either hot or cold.

Take a flowering spray of lemon verbena (with a few leaves) and put in a cup. Add boiling water and steep for 4 minutes, when the tisane should be a pale golden colour. Remove the flowers and foliage, and add a small dollop of honey, if desired.

lime blossom tisane

This pale yellow tisane has been used traditionally to promote a good night's sleep; it is surprisingly creamy.

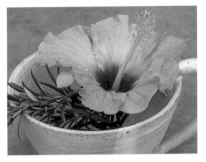

▲ Hibiscus flowers make a visual treat, as well as a soothing hot drink.

Pick lime flowers when they begin to open, using five or six for each cup. Add hot, not boiling, water and steep for 3–4 minutes. Remove the blossoms. Strain and drink with a slice of lemon.

hibiscus and rosemary tisane

With their flamboyant colouring, exotic hibiscus flowers make a dramatic and colourful tisane, enhanced with savoury rosemary.

Place one hibiscus flower and one rosemary sprig per cup and add some boiling water. Infuse for 4 minutes, removing the rosemary but leaving the hibiscus in place. Drink hot or chilled. Sweeten with honey.

▼ The fragrance of tisanes, such as lime blossom, acts as a mood enhancer.

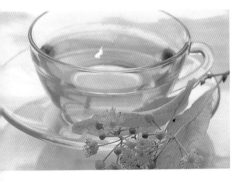

16 rejuvenating juices

Fresh fruit and vegetable juices play a vital role in detoxing – they stimulate the whole system and encourage the elimination of toxins. Drink juices fresh, as processing reduces nutritional values.

purple pep

For a healthy dose of antioxidants, try this rich, colourful juice.

3 carrots
115g/4 oz beetroot (beet)
30g/1 oz baby spinach
2 celery sticks

Scrub and trim the carrots and beetroot, then cut the beetroot into large chunks. Juice all the vegetables in a juice extractor, then pour into a glass and drink immediately.

citrus shake

This refreshing juice gently boosts the immune system.

1 pink grapefruit
1 blood orange
30ml/2 tbsp lemon juice

Peel the grapefruit and orange and cut into rough segments. Juice the fruit, then stir in the lemon juice.

juicing tips

• Drunk in the morning, fruit juices are useful for scouring waste products from the digestive tract.
•Vegetable juices are best drunk in the afternoon, as they re-establish the acid and alkaline balance of the body, giving a rejuvenating effect.
• Do not drink fresh juices if you suffer from health problems such as candida, diabetes or bowel disorders.

▼ *Purple Pep, an antioxidant powerhouse, and tangy and cleansing Citrus Shake.*

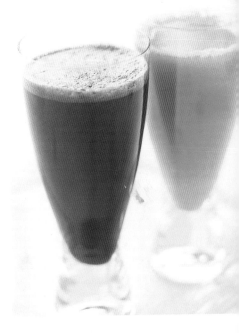

17

delicious smoothies

A blend of soft fruits and milk or yogurt, smoothies offer a tasty alternative to eating fruit. Their vitamin content makes them ideal detoxifiers. Summer smoothies can be partially frozen for a cool treat.

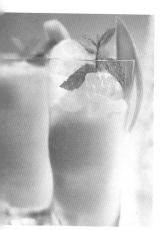

banana and mango smoothie

125g/4½oz banana
125g/4½oz mango
120ml/4fl oz/½ cup yogurt
   or milk

Peel and chop the banana and mango into large chunks. Place the fruit in a food processor or blender with the yogurt or milk. Process for 1–2 minutes, until smooth and creamy, and pour into a large glass.

Add a sprig of mint for a tasty bite.

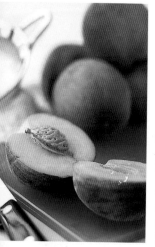

peach and blueberry smoothie

150g/5oz fresh peaches
150g/5oz blueberries
120ml/4fl oz/½ cup yogurt
   or milk

Stone (pit) the peaches and chop the flesh into large chunks. Drop the peaches and the blueberries into a blender and add the yogurt or milk. Process for 1–2 minutes until the mixture turns frothy, then pour into a large glass and serve.

Substitute raspberries or strawberries for the blueberries. Frozen berries may be used when fruit is out of season.

18

food & drinks to avoid

Diet is the key to a fit body and a lively mind. Poor eating habits suppress the body's efficiency, and the following should be excluded during detox – ideally, they should always be kept to a minimum.

processed foods

Many modern food production methods overprocess foods, leaving nutritional values diminished – fibre, minerals and vitamins are stripped away, and an excess of sugar, fats and salt are added. Commercial farming and storing methods also add harmful chemicals and preservatives. Buy fresh organic foods whenever possible.

alcohol

The occasional glass of wine does little harm, and may even help prevent heart disease. Drunk in large amounts, however, alcohol damages the liver, depletes vitamin stores and dehydrates the system.

caffeine

Found in coffee, tea, chocolate and soft drinks, caffeine is a powerful stimulant that raises blood pressure and exacerbates nervous conditions. Before starting a detox diet, reduce caffeine consumption gradually to avoid withdrawal symptoms.

dairy products

Butter, cheese and milk are high in unsaturated fats; these tend to slow down the lymphatic system, which is responsible for removing toxins from the body, so avoid when detoxing.

fish and meat

Meat is difficult to digest and, unless it is organic, may contain traces of growth hormones and preservatives used in production. Fish may contain pollutants, unless caught in deep seas.

salt and sugar

Excess salt overloads the kidneys and leads to water retention. Herbs or lemon juice are good substitutes. Refined sugars can upset the body's sugar balance. Natural sugars in fruits and honey are kinder on the system.

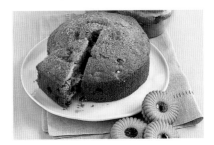

▸ *Eliminate cakes and biscuits, which are high in refined sugars, during a detox diet.*

mono-diet detox

Based on eating just one type of raw fruit or vegetable, a 1-day mono diet is an excellent introduction to detoxing that will have a noticeably positive effect on your health and vitality levels.

the diet

Choose one type of organic vegetable or ripe fresh fruit. You will need 1.6kg/3½ lb of either: grapes, apples, pears, pineapple, papaya, carrots, cucumber or celery. Eat small meals and vary the way you prepare the food. For example, you could grate your chosen fruit or vegetable for breakfast, juice it for lunch and eat it whole for dinner.

In the morning, drink a cup of hot water with the juice of a half a lemon to kick-start the liver. It is important to drink at least 1.5 litres/ 2½ pints/6¼ cups of still mineral water, or filtered tap water, at intervals throughout the day.

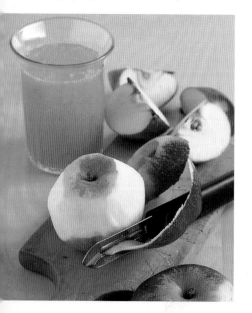

▼ After a 1-day mono diet, moving on to longer programmes will be simple.

vital exercise

• Morning: Practise simple stretches to stimulate your lymphatic system. Later in the morning, have an aromatherapy or a shiatsu massage, or try relaxation techniques such as deep breathing.

• Afternoon: Try some gentle yoga or Pilates exercises, or go for a swim, cycle or take a walk.

• Evening: Wind down by meditating or practising a simple visualization technique. Pamper yourself with a pedicure or manicure, read a book or listen to some calming music. Later, soak in an Epsom salts bath and prepare for bed early, perhaps relaxing with a good book or drinking a soothing herbal tea.

20

weekend detox

The 2-day detox plan is based on fruit and vegetable dishes and juices. Perfect for a quiet weekend, this is a gentle and effective detox that will give your digestive system a break.

the diet

• Morning: Kick-start your liver with a cup of hot water and lemon juice. For breakfast, prepare a fruit juice and dilute with water. Eat a small bunch of grapes or an apple mid-morning.

• Afternoon: Prepare a vegetable juice and a large salad for lunch, for example, tomatoes, cucumber, fennel, carrot and beetroot (beet). Drink plenty of water, either bottled mineral or filtered tap water.

• Evening: Have a dinner consisting of very lightly steamed vegetables, sprinkled with fresh herbs and lemon juice, along with some brown rice.

vital exercise

Take gentle exercise, such as yoga or Pilates, and do simple stretches all day. Walking or cycling will give you energy in the afternoon. It is a good idea to end each day with relaxation techniques or meditation.

don't detox:

• Directly after a bout of flu.

• If you have had liver disease or kidney failure; ask your doctor about diet.

• When under great stress; ie pressure at work, moving house, during a bereavement or after a divorce.

• If you have a serious medical condition or are taking prescription drugs for any reason.

• If you are pregnant or diabetic.

• If you are recovering from alcohol or drug addiction.

▼ *Eating mainly vegetables and fruit allows the body to focus on eliminating toxins.*

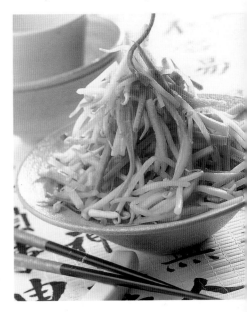

21

7-day detox

This rigorous plan is designed to provide a slow and steady detox. The plan combines and supplements the mono and weekend plans. Begin on a Friday, as the first few days are more intense.

the plan

• Day before: Ease into detox by including light, cleansing foods in your meals.

• Day one: Follow the guidelines for the 1-day mono diet.

• Days two and three: Follow the guidelines for the weekend detox. In the evening, have a sitz bath.

• Days four and five: Repeat days two and three, but include a fruit salad with yogurt for lunch and a baked potato with tofu or hummus for dinner. From day four, include snacks such as pumpkin seeds, dried fruit or nutty oat snack.

• Days six and seven: Repeat days four and five, including dried fruit steamed with fresh ginger. Add more protein to your meals, eg a grain or bean salad, lentil dahl or brown rice risotto. For dessert, eat live natural yogurt with a spoonful of honey. In the evening, take an Epsom salts bath to help flush out toxins.

• Days after: Slowly return to a healthy, varied diet based on nourishing, cleansing foods. Try not to overexert yourself, and avoid stressful situations, if at all possible.

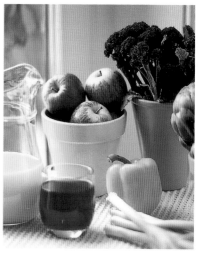

▲ The 7-day detox includes healthy, natural foods to help cleanse your system.

side effects

When following a detox programme, side effects are natural; their severity will depend on how many toxins are present in the system and how long your diet lasts. You may experience fatigue, headaches, nausea, chills, bad breath, furry tongue and irritability. Avoid painkillers; instead, drink plenty of water and herbal teas to aid the flushing out process.

22 hangover detox

If you have drunk too much alcohol, this hangover detox will ease the pain. The ideal is to consume a moderate amount in the first place, but the occasional overindulgence can be dealt with.

intake plan

Alcohol dehydrates your body, so keep sipping water all day. Although you may crave coffee and tea, caffeine acts as a diuretic – counter-productive when you are trying to rehydrate. Instead, try herbal teas with a little honey. To help settle your stomach and raise your blood sugar levels, eat a breakfast of natural muesli with yogurt and fruit, or a big bowl of porridge. For lunch, choose a light, filling meal that is low in fat – for example, a vegetable stir-fry with brown rice or couscous. At dinner time, a piece of baked fish or chicken with a salad, or a baked potato with salad are good choices.

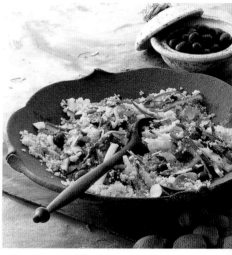

▲ *Prepare a low-fat nutritious lunch to settle your stomach and set you on the road to recovery.*

relax

You are bound to feel under par, so be kind to yourself. End the day with a relaxing bath; add several drops of lavender oil to help soothe you to sleep. By the next day, your body should be clear of the alcohol residue.

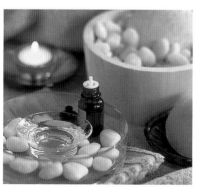

◀ *Try not to overtax your system when hungover – relax with some aromatherapy.*

23 aromatherapy oils

Aromatic essential oils are used in many ways to promote and restore health, as well as improve the quality of life with their scent. They are extracted from the flowers and foliage of plants and trees.

the oils

SANDALWOOD: A heavy-scented oil with antidepressant properties.

CHAMOMILE: This is a very relaxing, antispasmodic oil that relieves tension headaches and insomnia.

GERANIUM: This rose-scented oil has refreshing, antidepressant properties and is a very good treatment for nervousness and exhaustion.

BENZOIN: Vanilla-scented gum extract from an Asian tree. It is used in inhalation mixtures as it eases restricted breathing.

YLANG YLANG: This pungent oil is from an Indonesian tree and has a sedative, yet antidepressant action. It is good for panic attacks, insomnia, anxiety and depression.

PEPPERMINT: Its strong analgesic and antispasmodic properties make peppermint an ideal treatment for tension headaches.

EUCALYPTUS: One of the best oils for respiratory complaints.

JASMINE: A relaxing, euphoric aroma makes jasmine a great mood lifter.

LAVENDER: Useful for stress-related ailments, burns and skin care, lavender is one of the most versatile oils.

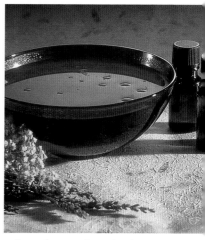

▲ Aromatherapy oils can be dispersed in a bowl of hot water or by using an oil burner.

FENNEL: One of the best detoxifying oils available.

ORANGE: An uplifting and detoxifying oil that helps to combat fluid retention and muscular aches and pains.

> Buy good-quality aromatherapy oils. Blend small amounts at a time, as their healing properties deteriorate when in contact with air. Store in a cool, dark place.

24 aromatherapy massage

A massage with aromatherapy oils is one of the most beneficial ways to ease tension, headaches and stress, and to help release toxins stored in body tissues and cells during a detox programme.

self-massage

Give yourself a break from work or an evening treat by using simple massage techniques. You can concentrate on one section of your body at a time, targetting tired and tense muscles. Choose a blend of essential oils – such as ylang ylang, orange and geranium – and add 1 per cent to a base oil, such as sweet almond or grapeseed oil.

with a partner

Massaging a partner is a great way to share physical contact, and relax and revive each other after a busy working day. Create a warm and comfortable space beforehand, using pillows or cushions for support, and cover his or her body with towels, if needed, to keep warm. Choose an oil blend that you both like, then warm the oil by rubbing it between your hands before applying to the skin.

You may want to light candles, as the diffused light will help you both relax. Calming New Age or classical music will help create a pleasant mood. After one partner has been massaged, you can swap places.

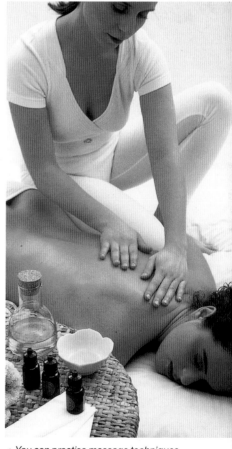

▲ You can practise massage techniques with a partner to boost energy levels.

25 face massage

The face collects tension during the day, and this simple massage can help you to unwind and prevent headaches from occurring. It also stimulates the circulation and lymph glands.

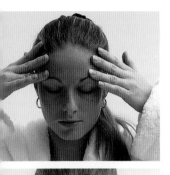

1 Starting in the centre of your forehead, make very small, circular movements with your fingertips and work slowly out towards the temples. Repeat three times.

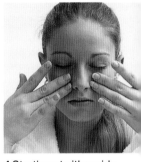

4 Starting at either side of your nose, move your fingers outwards using circular motions along the cheekbone to the jaw. Pay special attention to the jaw and chin area, where a lot of tension is held. Repeat five times.

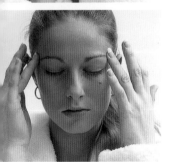

2 Use gentle finger movements to apply pressure to the area where the eye socket meets your nose. Repeat three times.

3 Move your fingers outwards along the brow bone from the top of your nose. Repeat this action five times.

FACE OIL
For a calming face massage, blend 4 drops of lavender and 2 drops of ylang ylang in a light oil, such as almond, grapeseed or coconut.

26 hand massage

For people who use computers, machinists and musicians, the hands may easily become strained through extended use. Regular breaks and self-massage can prevent repetitive strain injury.

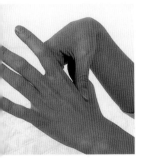

1 To release stored tensions and improve circulation, start by squeezing between each finger in turn, with the thumb and index finger of the other hand.

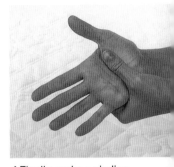

2 Make a rolling movement on each finger, slowly working your way from the knuckle to the fingertip, with firm pressure.

4 Finally, make a circling motion with one thumb on the palm of the other hand. This squeezes and stretches taut, contracted muscles. It should be a fairly deep action. Work all over the palm, maintaining a firm and even pressure.

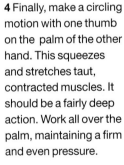

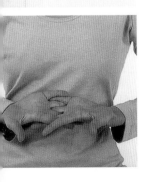

3 Stretch each digit with a gentle pulling action to ease tight tendons – there is no need to "crack" each finger. Interlock the fingers of both hands and stretch the palms.

Once you have completed steps 1 to 4, repeat each massage technique on the opposite hand.

27

neck & shoulder massage

Tense, aching muscles are often experienced in the neck and shoulders, causing head and back aches. Self-massage is very helpful in such cases, and it can be done anywhere.

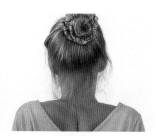

1 Begin by shrugging your shoulders, exaggerating their contraction by lifting them as far as possible, then letting them drop down and relax completely.

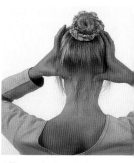

2 Firmly grip the opposite shoulder with your hand, and use a squeezing motion to loosen the tension. This "kneading" helps to remove waste matter from tired muscles and oxygenates the blood. Moving slowly around the shoulder, squeeze firmly. Repeat on the other side.

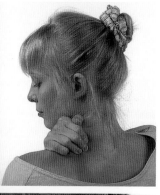

4 To work deeply into the neck, move the thumbs in a circular motion across the neck and up the base of the skull, using a moderate amount of pressure.

Self-massage of the shoulders and neck can be done anywhere, and without the need to get undressed. Release mounting tension in these areas before your shoulders become permanently hunched around your ears.

3 With the fingers of both hands, grip the back of your neck and squeeze in a circular motion to help relax the muscles leading up either side of the neck. Massage right up to the base of the skull, then down again to the base of the shoulders.

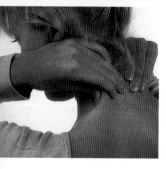

28 arm massage

The arms can feel sluggish by midday – especially if you are using your hands exclusively. This simple and effective routine will wake up tired muscles and joints, allowing the circulation to move again.

1 With one hand, perform a simple kneading action on the opposite arm. Squeeze up and down the arm rapidly, from the wrist to the shoulder and back again.

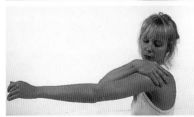

2 Knead more rapidly than in a normal massage. This will energize each arm and shoulder in turn.

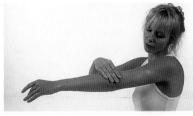

3 With your whole hand, rub the outside surface of the arm swiftly to stimulate the circulation.

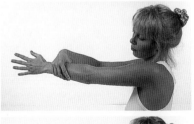

4 Repeat several times, in an upwards direction from your wrist to your shoulder, which will encourage blood to flow back to the heart.

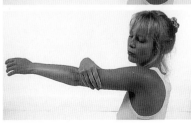

29 stomach & chest massage

Emotional tension is often stored in the torso – these bottled-up feelings may cause tight muscles across the chest and abdomen. Self-massage can help you release the stress.

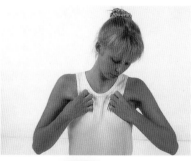

1 Using thumbs and fingers, grip your pectoral muscles on both sides of the chest leading towards the shoulders. Knead them firmly. If you have any tenderness in the breasts and lymph glands beneath the armpits (ie, women who are premenstrual), use a more gentle pressure.

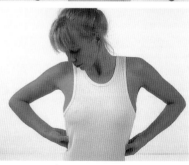

2 With a couple of fingers, feel in between the ribs for the intercostal muscles. Work firmly between each rib, moving the fingers in tiny circles. Repeat on each side.

3 Place your hands on your abdomen, and apply pressure slowly in a clockwise direction. Repeat a couple of times with increasing pressure, but ease off if this becomes painful – it is best not to overdo it. This action promotes digestive and bowel action.

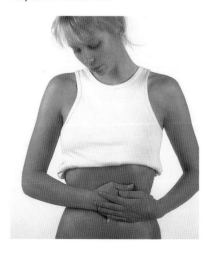

30 buttocks & thigh massage

For people whose jobs involve being on their feet all day, the thighs and buttocks can take a beating. This set of massage exercises will benefit aching muscles and restore circulation in swollen limbs.

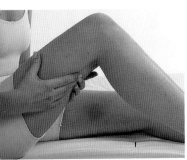

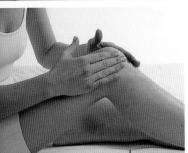

1 Start by working up the sides of the thighs. Using both hands, knead one thigh at a time, applying a firm pressure by squeezing muscles between the fingers and thumb.

2 Squeeze with each hand alternatively for the best effect, working from the front of the knee to the hip and back. Repeat on the other thigh.

3 Rising to a kneeling position, pummel your hips and buttocks, using a clenched fist and keeping your wrists flexible. This will get your circulation moving and also help to loosen cellulite in the tissues.

UPLIFTING OILS
Citrus oils have a tonic effect on the limbs; try adding a few drops of orange and lemon oil to a hot bath after your massage.

31 leg massage

Calves and knees may ache following physical exertion such as hiking, tennis, dancing and step and aerobic exercises. This massage sequence will allow your limbs to return to a neutral state.

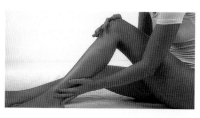

1 Sit in a comfortable position with one leg bent, so that you can easily reach down as far as your ankle.

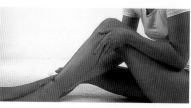

2 Stroke the leg lightly with both hands from ankle to thigh, repeating several times. Move the leg slightly each time to reach a different part. This will have a warming effect on the limbs.

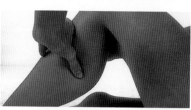

3 Using steady, firm pressure, work up the leg from ankle to knee with a squeezing action, paying particular attention to the back of the calves. This helps to move venous blood back towards the heart, and ease tension.

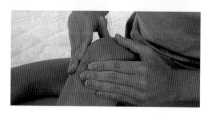

4 Massage the knee, slowly stroking around the outside of the kneecap, then use a circular pressure to move around the kneecaps more firmly with the fingertips.

32 foot massage

The feet are often ignored. Tight or ill-fitting shoes, jobs that require standing for hours on end, or strenuous dancing and sport all take their toll. This sequence will get your feet back into good shape.

1 Sit in a comfortable position so that you can easily reach a foot. Squeeze the foot, loosening up muscles and gently stretching the arch. Use firm pressure with your thumb to stretch the foot, then repeat on the other foot.

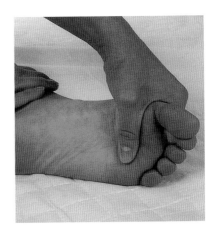

2 Now use small circular strokes to work all over the sole with your thumb. Pay special attention to the arch, working along the curve with your thumb. Now change or adjust your position, and work on the other foot in the same way.

If you prefer, massage the feet with 2-3 drops of a soothing aromatherapy oil, such as chamomile or jasmine, mixed in almond oil.

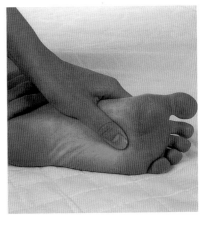

33 aerobic exercise

Aerobic exercises are those that raise the heart rate. Sustained by oxygen, they burn fat, boost the immune system and exercise the heart. Include them in detox to increase stamina and flexibility.

how to exercise

Walking, jogging, cycling and swimming all offer excellent aerobic exercise – with the bonus being that they are inexpensive and fun. Most gyms offer aerobics classes that use steps or weights, and these may be high or low impact. Choose a class that matches your fitness level. Dancing is another enjoyable way to exercise; many gyms offer classes in salsa, samba and ceroc, for example.

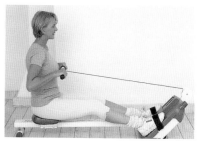

▲ Use simple exercise devices to get your aerobic activity during bad weather.

detox benefits

When following a detox plan, aerobics will help accelerate weight loss and eliminate toxins from the system. But go gently – you will not be consuming your usual amount of "fuel" in calories, so if you feel faint or light-headed, stop immediately. Remember to drink plenty of water.

stay motivated

Make exercise part of your daily routine by walking to work or on short journeys, such as collecting the children from school.

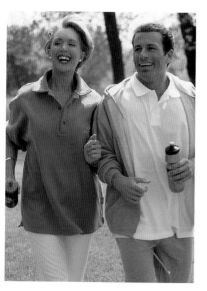

◀ Jogging or running with a friend is a pleasant way to stay motivated.

34   anaerobic exercise

During anaerobic exercise, the muscles work at high intensity for short bursts, and they become stronger with continued exercise. Try these arm exercises to allay back and shoulder problems.

arm lifts
Stand with your feet hip-width apart, keeping your knees soft and your spine straight. Take a weight in each hand, raise them above your head and circle your arms from the shoulder. Repeat the exercise five times.

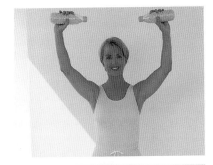

bicep curls
Hold weights down at your sides. Slowly bend your arms to bring the weights forwards and upwards, until they reach your shoulders. Repeat the exercise five times.

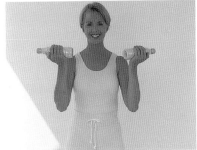

triceps
Place one hand on the back of a chair for support. Lean forwards, keeping your spine straight. Holding a weight at your side, slowly lift it behind you in a controlled movement. Repeat the movement five times, then do the exercise with the other arm.

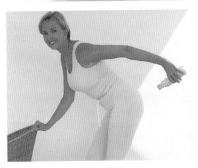

35 breathing

Under stress, we may breathe in a shallow way. This can lead to nervousness and panic attacks, as the system is starved of oxygen. Deep breathing oxygenates the blood, thus energizing the body.

deep breathing

Practising these exercises during detox will give you greater control over your breathing and help you to centre your thoughts, allowing you to focus on your goals. You can use them at work, at home or any time to invoke a feeling of peacefulness.

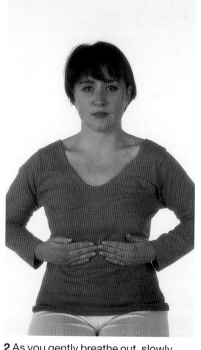

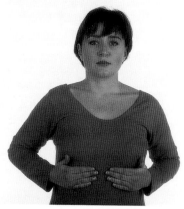

1 Place your hands just below the breastbone and take slow, deep breaths. As you breathe in, push out your stomach. This should make your hands move apart a little, and indicates that the diaphragm is moving as it should.

2 As you gently breathe out, slowly pull in your stomach muscles. Your diaphragm will move back upwards, and your hands will come together again. Repeat this exercise three or four times, and then begin to breathe normally again.

36 meditation

With so many activities, cares and responsibilities packed into a day, it is easy to feel overwhelmed. Meditation helps calm the mind, enabling you to approach tasks feeling balanced and refreshed.

prepare to meditate

Set aside a quiet place, perhaps lighting a candle or burning incense. You can sit cross-legged on a cushion, or recline on a bed or sofa. The following meditation can be recorded on tape if you find it helpful to listen to the sound of the words.

the haven

In this meditation, you will find your own special place – real or imaginary – in which to rest and feel safe. Close your eyes and allow your mind to drift. Where is this special place?

It may be a place you visited as a child, in a quiet corner of a wood or a secret room in a ruined castle, where you found yourself suddenly away from other people. Go to the place ... feel what made it special ... what makes it special still ... it belongs only to you, so you can think and do whatever you like ...

Notice what sort of light shines in through the branches outside the window ... is it bright or hazy? ... Does the temperature feel soothingly warm or refreshingly cool? ... Be aware of the colours that surround

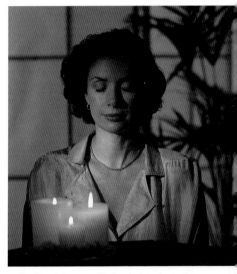

▲ During detox, meditation helps cleanse the mind of debris, as well as the body.

you ... the outlines of shapes ... the textures ... What sounds do you hear? ... Distant voices, church bells or perhaps birds singing ...

No one is asking anything of you ... no one expects anything of you ... you don't need to be anywhere ... except here, a place where everything is peaceful and you can truly relax and let yourself go ...

37 visualization

Simple visualization techniques can help you cope with stress. By letting your imagination "see" beyond the current crisis, you can register new ideas and ways of dealing with difficult people and situations.

the protective bubble

Imagine that you are in a situation that has, in the past, made you feel anxious. Picture the location and the people involved. See yourself there with them ... and notice a slight shimmer of light surrounding you, a sort of glowing "bubble" between you and the other people ... a protective bubble that reflects any negative feelings back on to them, leaving you the space to get on with your work, your life and developing your inner strength and calmness.

Concentrate on the bubble that surrounds and protects you at all times. It will only allow positive feelings to pass through, for you to enjoy and build upon. Others may feel negativity, but you are protected ... you can deal with whatever comes across your path in a calm and clear way. You are able to see the way forward ... solve problems ... find your way around difficulties ... by using your own rich inner resources and talents.

Imagine pushing out through the bubble emotions that are unhelpful ... such as jealousy, embarrassments, past resentments ... Push them out to where they can no longer harm or hinder you. Now you can keep things in better perspective, accepting the things you cannot change. You can control the way you think and act ... how you deal with others ... and move on with confidence and happiness.

◄ *Visualizations to improve your overall confidence levels can act as a rehearsal for future situations.*

38 stretches

When the limbs become tired, through tension or fatigue, the contraction of the muscles can lead to poor circulation. A few simple stretches can help restore the blood supply and relieve tight muscles.

blood flow enhancer

Chronic stress can make you feel tight across the chest and make your hands feel cold. This exercise will facilitate blood flow, allowing you to breathe more deeply, which will nourish all the cells in the body and warm the extremities.

Practise simple stretching exercises during detox to help release toxins from the tissues.

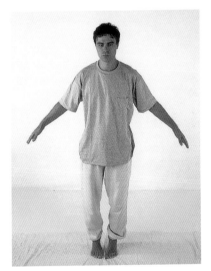

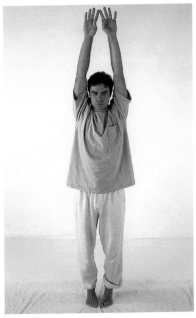

1 Stand with your feet close together and your arms resting by your sides. Slowly take a deep breath in, and at the same time, raise your arms out to your sides. Rise up on your toes.

2 Raise your arms until they meet directly over your head. As you exhale, slowly return to the original position. Repeat the sequence just three or four times more.

After a **warm** bath, take a brief **icy-cold** shower or bath to boost the circulation and encourage the removal of **toxins**.

40 salt bath

A bath with Epsom salts will help to eliminate toxins from the skin by drawing out impurities, leaving your body feeling wonderfully smooth and firm. Use during the 7-day detox.

taking a salt bath

As you run warm water into the bath, pour 450g/1lb of Epsom salts under the tap, so that they dissolve and disperse. Lie back in a comfortable position for 20 minutes, adding more hot water if the bath becomes too cool.

Afterwards, pat your skin dry, wrap yourself up in a warm towel and relax for an hour, or go to bed. You may sweat during the night, so drink plenty of water before you go to sleep and plenty in the morning. When you wake, take a normal bath or shower to remove any salty residues.

> **CAUTION**
> • If you suffer from high blood pressure, it is best to avoid the Epsom salts bath.

▾ Epsom salts are very high in magnesium, a soothing balm for tired, aching muscles.

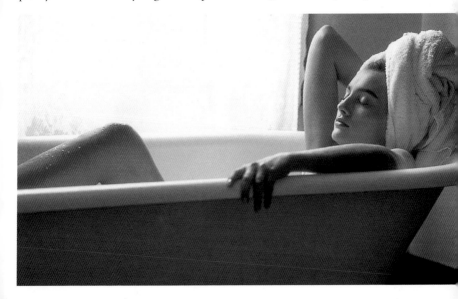

41

body scrub

Although fairly new in the West, body scrubs have been a Middle Eastern tradition for centuries. Use a body scrub whenever you feel the need for a deep cleanse that will promote good circulation.

citrus body scrub

The slightly gritty texture of this freshly scented exfoliating scrub helps to remove dead skin cells and stimulates the blood supply, leaving your skin feeling tingling and well toned. The recipe makes enough for five treatments.

45ml/3 tbsp ground sunflower seeds
45ml/3 tbsp medium oatmeal
45ml/3 tbsp flaked sea salt
45ml/3 tbsp grated orange peel
15ml/1 tbsp grated lemon peel
3 drops grapefruit essential oil
glass jar with lid
almond oil

Mix all the ingredients thoroughly and store in the sealed glass jar. When ready for a treatment, make a paste with ⅕ of the scrub and some almond oil in a shallow bowl. Remove all your clothes and stand in the bath. Gently massage the scrub all over your body, paying particular attention to areas of hard, dry skin such as the elbows, knees and ankles. Remove the residue before showering or bathing.

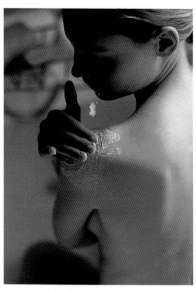

▲ An exfoliating body scrub will leave your skin glowing and healthy.

• Use a body scrub before moisturizing your skin and before applying tanning lotion.

• Body scrubs are a perfect way to perk up winter skin during dark, cold months when it does not receive much sunshine.

42 skin brushing

Brushing the skin with a dry, natural bristle brush is an exhilarating way to boost your circulation. Not only does it make your skin feel smooth, it stimulates the senses and helps to eliminate cellulite.

10-minute routine

The whole process of skin brushing should take about 10 minutes – this is plenty of time to go over your entire body. Try brushing in the morning before taking a bath or shower. Skin brushing will also help the effectiveness of an aromatherapy bath, making your skin and pores more open to the oils.

HOW TO BRUSH SKIN

1 Start with your feet and toes. Using long strokes (towards your heart), brush up the front and back of your legs. Move up to your thighs and groin area.

2 Brush over your buttocks, up to the lower back.

3 Now brush gently along your hands and arms, inwards towards the heart.

4 Gently brush your stomach, using circular, clockwise motions.

5 Move across your shoulders, down over your chest (lightly over the breasts). Finally, move down your back, towards your heart.

▸ *For super-soft skin, brush gently with a sisal mitt or brush in the bath or shower.*

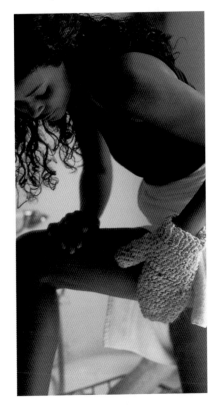

43 saunas & steam baths

Traditionally, hot dry or steam baths have been utilized by many peoples, from Scandinavians to Native Americans. They have the power to purify body, mind and soul.

a detox bath

Saunas and steam baths work by encouraging perspiration (sweat) and boosting the circulation, which in turn help eliminate toxins from the system. It is best to spend between 5–10 minutes in the heat at a time, then take a cold shower or swim in between. Finish your session with a cold shower, then relax for 30 minutes until your body has adjusted to its normal temperature.

CAUTION

• If you suffer from heart problems or high blood pressure, avoid saunas and steam baths.

• It is a good idea to abstain from eating heavy meals, or drinking alcohol and caffeine before taking a sauna or steam bath.

▾ You can use the time after a cleansing sauna or steam bath to relax and meditate.

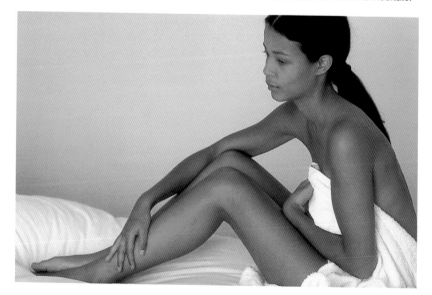

44 mud wrap

The healing properties of mud are well known around the world. When used as a skin wrap, its high mineral content nourishes the body, heals wounds, clears rashes and reduces cellulite.

spa treatment

The best way to get a full mud wrap is to pamper yourself and visit one of the many spas that offer the treatment. A special mud – which may also contain herbs and spices – is smeared all over your body; following this, you are wrapped in a plastic sheet. Towels are wrapped around you to keep your body temperature even while the mud works to draw out impurities. After perspiring gently for about 20 minutes, you can take a shower, pat yourself dry and then luxuriate in the smooth and clean texture of your skin.

types of mud

Mud wraps use various types of local mud, each of which has its own special properties. White Thai mud, also called *din so porng*, is mixed with turmeric, marjoram and spring water – it has antiperspirant, coolant and moisturizing properties. In Northern California, a local mud mixed with crushed Napa Valley grape seeds purifies and tones the skin, while Moor mud, which is rich in black magma, minerals, amino antibodies

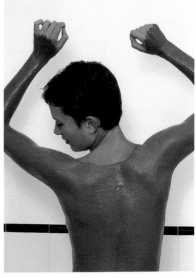

▲ *Ideal for detoxing, mud wraps work from the outside-in to promote good health.*

and salicylic acid (the substance used in aspirin) relieves rheumatic aches and injuries.

Mud face masks promote a glowing complexion and are easy to use at home.

45

face scrub

The face is subject to the ill effects of weather, pollution and often alcohol and cigarette smoke. Exfoliating delicate tissues with a gentle face scrub will leave your skin feeling soft and renewed.

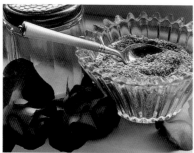

Treat yourself to the following all-natural, rose-scented face scrub. It is best to choose pure, organic ingredients; these will be readily available from many supermarkets and health food stores. You can purchase the rose petals from a herbalist – or pick, dry and powder blooms from your own garden. This recipe makes enough for about ten treatments.

cleopatra face scrub
45ml/3 tbsp ground almonds
45ml/3 tbsp medium oatmeal
45ml/3 tbsp powdered milk
30ml/2 tbsp powdered rose petals
glass jar with lid
almond oil

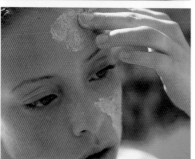

Mix all the dry ingredients together in the jar. Before using, mix a small portion with almond oil to form a soft paste. With the lightest touch, rub the mixture into your skin, using a gentle circular motion. Be careful to avoid the delicate area around your eyes. Finally, rinse off the face scrub with warm water and pat your face dry with a soft towel.

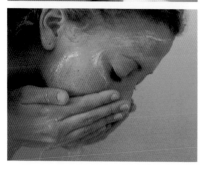

46 steam facial

Steam facials open the pores and deep-clean the skin: the heat relaxes the pores and boosts blood circulation. With the addition of herbs and flowers, the stimulating and cleansing action is magnified.

rose and chamomile facial

Fill a bowl just wider than your face with hot water, and add 3 drops of rose essential oil and 4 drops of chamomile essential oil. Cover your head with a towel, draping it over the bowl. Let steam waft over your face for 5 minutes, then relax in a quiet place for a further 15 minutes before closing the pores.

Dab cooled skin with one of the following toners: for dry skin, mix 75ml/5 tbsp triple-distilled rose water with 30ml/2 tbsp orange flower water. Oily skins should use 90ml/6 tbsp rose water mixed with 30ml/2 tbsp witch hazel. Store concoctions in clean bottles and keep cool or refrigerate.

fresh facials

Instead of using essential oils, float fresh flowers and leaves, such as chamomile or rose petals, in hot water. You could also try mint, marjoram, lavender or marigold.

> **CAUTION**
> Do not use a steam facial if you are prone to thread veins.

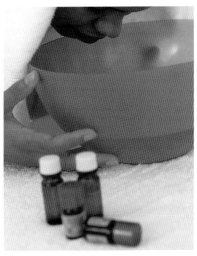

▲ After an aromatherapy facial, you will be confident that your skin looks its best.

▼ The power of a flower's scent leaves you feeling refreshed and rejuvenated.

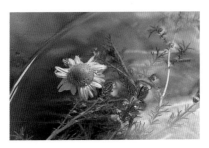

mouth cleansing

The mouth is an area where cleanliness is particularly important. Many herbs can be used to keep the breath fresh and the teeth white – you can make your own natural mixtures for oral hygiene.

sage-and-salt tooth powder
25g/1oz fresh sage leaves
60ml/4 tbsp sea salt

With a pair of scissors, shred the sage leaves finely and scatter them into an ovenproof dish. Grind the sea salt into the leaves with a wooden spoon or pestle. Bake the ground mixture at 140°C/275°F/Gas 1 for about 1 hour, until the sage is dry and crisp. Pound it down again until it is reduced to a powder. Use the powder on a damp toothbrush instead of toothpaste.

spicy lemon verbena mouthwash
5ml/1 tsp each ground nutmeg,
    ground cloves, cardamom pods
    and caraway seeds
small handful fresh lemon verbena
    leaves or 15g/½ oz dried verbena
600ml/1 pint/2½ cups purified water
30ml/2 tbsp sweet sherry

Simmer the spices, lemon verbena and water in a pan for 30 minutes. Strain through a sieve. Add sherry and pour into a clean bottle. To use, dilute 15-30ml/1-2 tbsp in a glass of water.

SIMPLE BREATH FRESHENERS
• Chew the fresh-picked leaves of parsley, watercress or mint after eating a meal with garlic or onions.
• Suck or chew on fennel and caraway seeds, star anise, angelica or cloves.
• Dilute half-and-half rose water with mineral water and use the mixture as a mouthrinse.

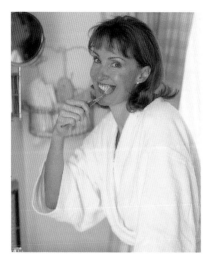

◀ *A glowing smile and fresh breath are not only attractive, they signal good health.*

48 hair detox

Many people wash, condition and style too often, resulting in a build-up of commercial products that contain chemicals and additives. Give your hair a detox treat by making your own herbal hair rinses.

Make up one of these fresh rinses in a jug before you begin washing. Hold your head over a bowl as you pour the herbal rinse through your hair, then pour back the rinse from the bowl to the jug. Re-apply at least five times for really shiny hair.

rosemary rinse for dark hair
40g/1½ oz fresh rosemary sprigs
1 litre/1¾ pints/4 cups boiling water

Put the sprigs in a jug and pour in the boiling water. Leave to stand and steep for 1 hour, then strain off the herbs through a sieve. Because of the high essential oil content of rosemary, the rinse is also good for dry hair.

chamomile rinse for fair hair
25g/1oz dried chamomile flowers or 40g/1½oz fresh flowers and leaves
1 litre/1¾pints/4 cups boiling water

Prepare and use this rinse in the same way as the dark hair rosemary rinse described above.

▸ *Natural hair rinses are inexpensive and will keep your locks healthy and shiny.*

nettle rinse for dandruff
1 litre/1¾ pints/4 cups boiling water
25g/1oz fresh nettle leaves
25g/1oz nasturtium flowers
30ml/2 tbsp cider vinegar
30ml/2 tbsp witch hazel

Pour the water over the nettles and nasturtiums (nettles lose their sting in boiling water). Leave to stand overnight, then strain off the herbs, and add vinegar and witch hazel. Pour through as a final rinse every time you shampoo.

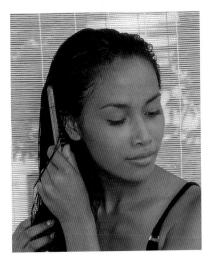

49 foot soaks

Soaking the feet in a hot, invigorating bath not only thoroughly refreshes your feet, but it can lift your mood as well: the warmth relaxes your body and the soothing herbs calm your mind.

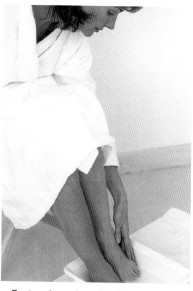

▲ Foot soaks are beneficial during detox – they also soothe colds, flu or chills.

mustard foot bath

15ml/1 tbsp mustard powder
2.2 litres/4 pints/9 cups hot water

Stir the mustard into the water until it is dissolved. Immerse the feet while the bath is still hot. Reheat if required.

▶ A foot bath revitalizes the whole body.

herb foot bath for aching feet

50g/2oz mixed fresh herbs:
    peppermint, yarrow, pine needles,
    chamomile flowers, rosemary
1 litre/1¾ pints/4 cups boiling water
1.75 litres/3 pints/7½ cups hot water
15ml/1 tbsp borax
15ml/1 tbsp Epsom salts

Roughly chop the herbs, place into a large bowl and pour in the boiling water. Leave to stand for 1 hour. Strain, and add to a basin containing the hot water; the final temperature of the foot bath should be comfortably warm. Stir in the borax and Epsom salts, immerse your feet and soak for 15–20 minutes.

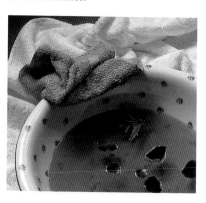

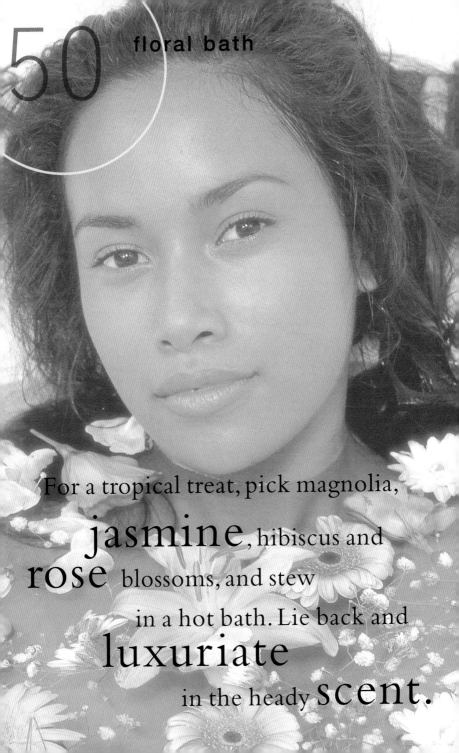

For a tropical treat, pick magnolia, jasmine, hibiscus and rose blossoms, and stew in a hot bath. Lie back and luxuriate in the heady scent.

index

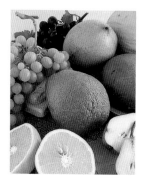
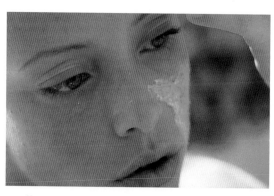

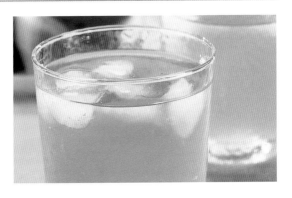

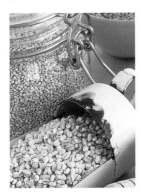

This edition is published by Lorenz Books, an imprint of Anness Publishing Ltd, Blaby Road, Wigston, Leicestershire LE18 4SE; info@anness.com

www.lorenzbooks.com; www.annesspublishing.com

If you like the images in this book and would like to investigate using them for publishing, promotions or advertising, please visit our website www.practicalpictures.com for more information.

© Anness Publishing Ltd 2013

A CIP catalogue record for this book is available from the British Library

Publisher: Joanna Lorenz
Managing editor: Helen Sudell
Editor: Melanie Halton
Design: Jester Designs
Photography: Sue Atkinson, Steve Baxter, Simon Bottomley, Martin Brigdale, Nick Cole, Nicky Dowey, James Duncan, Gus Filgate, John Freeman, Ian Garlick, Michelle Garrett, Amanda Heywood, Janine Hosegood, Alistair Hughes, Dave Jordan, Dave King, Don Last, William Lingwood, Lucy Mason, Liz McAuley, Thomas Odulate, Debbie Patterson, Fiona Pragoff, Craig Robertson, Carin Simon, Sam Stowell.
Production controller: Wendy Lawson
Indexer: Hilary Bird

PUBLISHER'S NOTE

Although the advice and information in this book are believed to be accurate and true at the time of going to press, neither the authors nor the publisher can accept any legal responsibility or liability for any errors or omissions that may have been made nor for any inaccuracies nor for any loss, harm or injury that comes about from following instructions or advice in this book.

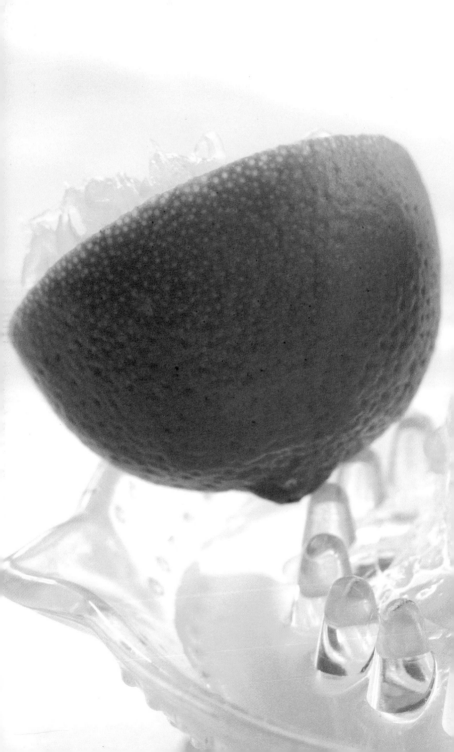